PREGNANCY GUIDE

For First Time Dads

Navigating New Fatherhood:
Your Essential Companion
Through Pregnancy

Sandra Morgan

TABLE OF CONTENTS

INTRODUCTION

Pregnancy Guide for First-Time Dads
Becoming a father for the first time is an exhilarating experience, filled with excitement, anticipation, and perhaps a touch of nervousness. As your partner embarks on the incredible journey of pregnancy, you, too, are about to embark on a transformative journey—one that will shape your life in profound ways. While much of the focus during pregnancy naturally falls on the expectant mother, the role of the father is equally crucial. As a first-time dad, your support, understanding, and involvement can make all the difference in your partner's pregnancy experience.

Understanding Pregnancy
Before diving into the specifics of supporting your partner during pregnancy, it's essential to gain a basic understanding of what she's going through. Pregnancy is a complex biological process that lasts approximately 40 weeks, divided into three trimesters. Each trimester brings its own set of physical and emotional changes for both the mother and the baby.

During the first trimester, your partner may experience symptoms such as morning sickness, fatigue, and mood swings as her body adjusts to the hormonal changes. The second trimester is often referred to as the "honeymoon phase" of pregnancy, characterized by reduced symptoms and the beginnings of feeling the baby's movements. The third trimester brings its own challenges, including increased discomfort, nesting instincts, and anticipation for the arrival of the baby.

Your Role as a Supportive Partner
As a first-time dad, your role as a supportive partner is invaluable. Your presence, reassurance, and involvement can greatly contribute to your partner's well-being throughout the pregnancy journey. Here are some essential ways you can support her:

1. Educate Yourself
Take the time to educate yourself about pregnancy, childbirth, and newborn care. Understanding the process will not only help you support your partner better but also alleviate any anxieties you may have about becoming a father.

2. Attend Prenatal Appointments
Accompany your partner to prenatal appointments whenever possible. This will not only strengthen your bond as a couple but also allow you to be actively involved in your baby's healthcare journey.

3. Be Empathetic
 Pregnancy can be physically and emotionally demanding for your partner. Be empathetic, patient, and understanding of her needs, and offer your support in any way you can.

4. Be Involved
Get involved in the pregnancy experience by
participating in decision-making processes, setting
up the nursery, and attending childbirth education
classes together. Your active involvement will make
your partner feel supported and valued.

5. Take Care of Yourself
While supporting your partner is crucial, don't forget
to take care of yourself as well. Maintain a healthy
lifestyle, communicate openly with your partner
about your feelings, and seek support from friends,
family, or a therapist if needed.

Becoming a father for the first time is a remarkable
journey filled with joy, anticipation, and
responsibility. By understanding the intricacies of
pregnancy and actively supporting your partner
every step of the way, you can strengthen your
bond as a couple and prepare for the arrival of your
little one with confidence and excitement. Embrace
the journey ahead with an open heart and a
willingness to learn, grow, and cherish every
moment of this extraordinary experience.

Why this book is for you

This book, "Pregnancy Guide for First-Time Dads,"
is specifically crafted with you in mind because it
acknowledges the unique and pivotal role you play
as a first-time father during this transformative

journey. Here's why this book is tailored to meet your needs:

Comprehensive Guidance: As a first-time dad, you may feel overwhelmed by the prospect of supporting your partner through pregnancy. This guide provides comprehensive information on every aspect of pregnancy, childbirth, and newborn care, empowering you with the knowledge and confidence to navigate this journey alongside your partner.

Practical Advice: From attending prenatal appointments to setting up the nursery, this book offers practical advice on how you can actively participate in the pregnancy experience. It provides actionable steps and tips to help you support your partner effectively and be an involved father from the very beginning.

Emotional Support: Pregnancy can be a rollercoaster of emotions for both you and your partner. This book recognizes the emotional challenges you may face as a first-time dad and offers empathetic guidance on how to navigate these feelings. Whether you're experiencing anxiety, excitement, or uncertainty, this book provides reassurance and understanding.

Inclusive Perspective: While pregnancy is often portrayed as solely the mother's experience, this book emphasizes the importance of your role as a father. It celebrates the bond between you and your partner as equal partners in this journey and encourages your active involvement every step of the way.

Preparation for Parenthood: Beyond pregnancy, this book prepares you for the transition into parenthood. It covers topics such as newborn care, adjusting to life with a baby, and maintaining a healthy relationship with your partner postpartum. By equipping you with the necessary skills and knowledge, this book sets you up for success as a new parent.

Encouragement and Inspiration: Becoming a father for the first time is a momentous occasion, and this book celebrates the joys and wonders of fatherhood. It offers encouragement, inspiration, and anecdotes from real-life first-time dads, reminding you that you're not alone in this journey and that fatherhood is a deeply rewarding experience.

Overall, "Pregnancy Guide for First-Time Dads" is a comprehensive, practical, and empathetic resource designed to support you through one of the most significant transitions in your life. Whether you're feeling excited, nervous, or somewhere in between, this book is here to guide you with warmth, understanding, and expert advice every step of the way.

What to expect from pregnancy and parenthood

Expecting a child is an extraordinary journey filled with anticipation, excitement, and a multitude of changes, both anticipated and unexpected. Understanding what to expect from pregnancy and parenthood can help you navigate this transformative experience with confidence and readiness.

Pregnancy:

Physical Changes:
First Trimester: Your partner may experience symptoms such as morning sickness, fatigue, and mood swings as her body adjusts to hormonal changes.
Second Trimester: Often considered the "honeymoon phase," symptoms may subside, and your partner may start to feel the baby's movements.
Third Trimester: Your partner's body undergoes significant changes as the baby grows, leading to increased discomfort, nesting instincts, and anticipation for the baby's arrival.
Emotional Rollercoaster:
Pregnancy hormones can cause mood swings and emotional fluctuations for both you and your partner. It's essential to communicate openly and support each other through these changes.

Prenatal Care:
Regular prenatal appointments are crucial for monitoring the health of both your partner and the baby. These appointments include check-ups, ultrasounds, and discussions about birth plans and parenting choices.

Lifestyle Adjustments:
Your lifestyle may need to adapt to accommodate your partner's pregnancy, including dietary changes, avoiding certain activities or substances, and creating a supportive environment at home.

Parenthood:

Sleep Deprivation:
Newborns require frequent feeding and care, leading to disrupted sleep patterns for both parents. Expect to be sleep-deprived in the early months of parenthood.

Learning Curve:
Parenthood comes with a steep learning curve as you navigate feeding, diapering, soothing techniques, and understanding your baby's cues. Be patient with yourself and each other as you adjust to your new roles.

Emotional Rollercoaster:
Parenthood brings a range of emotions, from overwhelming love and joy to moments of doubt, worry, and exhaustion. It's normal to experience a mix of emotions as you bond with your baby and adjust to your new life.

Support System:
Building a support system of family, friends, and healthcare professionals can provide invaluable

assistance and guidance as you navigate parenthood. Don't hesitate to lean on others for support when needed.

Bonding and Connection:

Parenthood offers countless opportunities for bonding and connection with your baby. Whether through feeding, cuddling, or playing, cherish these moments and nurture your relationship with your child.

Growth and Development:

Parenthood is a journey of continuous growth and development, both for you as a parent and for your child. Embrace the challenges and joys of each stage of your child's development, from infancy through childhood and beyond.

In summary, pregnancy and parenthood are profound experiences filled with changes, challenges, and moments of unparalleled joy. By understanding what to expect and embracing the journey with an open heart and a willingness to learn, grow, and adapt, you can navigate this extraordinary chapter of life with confidence and grace.

How to support your partner and yourself

Supporting your partner and yourself during pregnancy and parenthood is essential for maintaining physical and emotional well-being, strengthening your relationship, and nurturing a positive environment for your growing family. Here are some elaborate ways to provide support:

Supporting Your Partner:

1. Emotional Support:
Be Present: Listen attentively to your partner's concerns, fears, and joys. Offer empathy, understanding, and validation of her experiences.
Encourage Open Communication: Create a safe space for your partner to express her emotions openly without fear of judgment.
Affirmation and Encouragement: Offer words of affirmation and encouragement to boost her confidence and reassure her of your love and support.

2. Practical Support:
Assist with Daily Tasks: Help out with household chores, cooking, and running errands to alleviate your partner's physical burden.
Attend Prenatal Appointments: Accompany your partner to prenatal appointments whenever possible to show your involvement and support.
Research and Educate Yourself: Take the initiative to learn about pregnancy, childbirth, and newborn care to better support your partner through this journey.

3. Physical Support:
Provide Physical Comfort: Offer massages, assist with stretches, and provide pillows or cushions for

your partner's comfort, especially during the later stages of pregnancy.

Be Flexible and Patient: Understand that your partner's physical needs and limitations may change throughout pregnancy. Adapt and accommodate as needed.

4. Encourage Self-Care:

Prioritize Rest: Encourage your partner to rest and take breaks when needed. Offer to take on extra responsibilities to allow her time to relax.

Promote Healthy Habits: Support your partner in maintaining a balanced diet, staying hydrated, and engaging in gentle exercise suitable for pregnancy.

Plan Relaxing Activities: Schedule leisure activities or pampering sessions to help your partner unwind and de-stress.

Supporting Yourself:

1. Self-Care:

Prioritize Your Needs: Take time for self-care activities that rejuvenate and replenish your energy, whether it's exercising, reading, or spending time with friends.

Seek Support: Don't hesitate to lean on your own support network of friends, family, or support groups for guidance and encouragement.

Practice Stress Management: Implement stress-reduction techniques such as deep breathing, meditation, or mindfulness to manage the challenges of pregnancy and parenthood.

2. Maintain Communication:
Express Your Feelings: Share your thoughts, concerns, and aspirations with your partner openly and honestly. Communication is key to strengthening your relationship and navigating parenthood together.
Address Concerns Promptly: If you're feeling overwhelmed or anxious, address your concerns with your partner and seek professional support if needed.

3. Bond with Your Baby:
Participate in Pregnancy Activities: Attend childbirth education classes, read books on parenting, and engage in bonding activities such as talking or singing to your baby bump.
Prepare for Parenthood: Take an active role in preparing for the arrival of your baby by setting up the nursery, assembling baby gear, and participating in parenting discussions with your partner.

4. Nurture Your Relationship:
Make Time for Each Other: Prioritize quality time together as a couple, whether it's through date nights, walks, or simple moments of connection.
Express Appreciation: Show gratitude for your partner's support and efforts, and express your love and appreciation regularly.
By prioritizing support for both your partner and yourself, you can create a nurturing and loving

environment that fosters mutual growth, resilience, and joy as you embark on the journey of pregnancy and parenthood together.

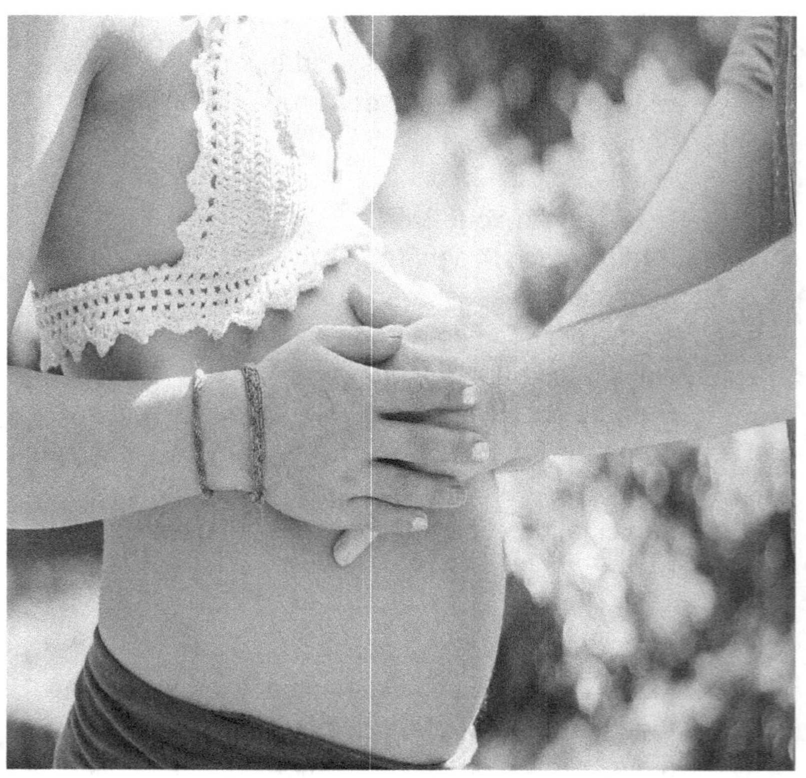

The First Trimester

Baby development: what's happening during the first trimester[1]

During the first trimester of pregnancy, which spans from week 1 to week 12, remarkable developments occur as the fertilized egg transforms into a recognizable human form. Here's a comprehensive overview of what happens during this crucial period:

Fertilization and Implantation: The first trimester begins with fertilization, where the sperm penetrates the egg, forming a zygote. As it travels down the fallopian tube towards the uterus, the zygote divides rapidly. Around day 6-7 after fertilization, the embryo implants itself into the uterine lining, initiating pregnancy.

Formation of the Embryo: By the end of the first month, the embryo has developed three distinct layers: the ectoderm, endoderm, and mesoderm, which will eventually give rise to all the body's organs and tissues.

Organogenesis: During weeks 4 to 8, organogenesis takes place, where major organs and structures begin to form. The neural tube, which eventually develops into the brain and spinal cord, closes during this time. The heart begins to beat and can often be detected via ultrasound around week 6. Limb buds emerge, and facial features start to take shape.

Development of Body Systems: By week 12, the basic structures of the respiratory, digestive, and circulatory systems are in place, although they are not yet fully functional. The placenta, a vital organ for nutrient exchange between the mother and fetus, also develops during this time.

Maternal Changes: Alongside fetal development, significant changes occur in the mother's body during the first trimester. Hormonal shifts can lead to symptoms such as morning sickness, fatigue, breast tenderness, and mood swings. The uterus expands to accommodate the growing embryo, leading to cramping and stretching sensations.

Confirmation of Pregnancy: During the first trimester, many women confirm their pregnancies through home pregnancy tests or clinical tests that detect human chorionic gonadotropin (hCG), a hormone produced by the placenta.

Risk of Miscarriage: Unfortunately, the first trimester also carries the highest risk of miscarriage, especially during the early weeks when fetal development is most vulnerable. Genetic abnormalities or developmental issues can sometimes lead to spontaneous abortion.

Prenatal Care: Prenatal care is crucial during the first trimester to monitor the health of both the mother and the developing fetus. This includes regular check-ups with healthcare providers, prenatal vitamins, and screening tests for genetic disorders or other complications.

Overall, the first trimester lays the foundation for the entire pregnancy, with rapid and intricate developments occurring as the embryo transforms into a fetus. While it is a period of excitement and anticipation for expecting parents, it also requires vigilance and care to ensure a healthy outcome for both mother and baby.

Pregnancy symptoms: what your partner may experience and how to help

During pregnancy, partners often experience a range of physical and emotional symptoms alongside the expecting mother. Understanding these symptoms and providing support can strengthen the bond between partners and make the pregnancy journey more manageable. Here's a comprehensive overview:

Morning Sickness: Nausea and vomiting, commonly referred to as morning sickness, can affect partners just as it does pregnant individuals. Offer support by preparing bland snacks, accompanying them to appointments, and helping with household chores when they're feeling unwell.

Fatigue: Pregnancy-related fatigue can be overwhelming, making it challenging for partners to maintain their usual energy levels. Encourage rest, assist with tasks, and be understanding if they need to take breaks or modify their activities.

Mood Swings: Hormonal fluctuations during pregnancy can lead to mood swings and emotional sensitivity. Practice patience, active listening, and provide reassurance during times of heightened emotions. Encourage open communication and be willing to discuss any concerns or fears they may have.

Food Aversions and Cravings: Partners may also experience changes in their appetite, including food aversions and cravings. Be flexible with meal planning, accommodate their dietary preferences, and be supportive of their cravings, even if they seem unusual.

Body Changes: Pregnancy can cause physical changes in partners, such as weight gain, breast tenderness, and skin changes. Offer compliments and reassurance about their appearance, and encourage them to prioritize self-care activities like gentle exercise and skincare routines.

Anxiety and Stress: It's common for partners to experience anxiety and stress about the pregnancy, childbirth, and parenthood. Listen actively, provide emotional support, and offer to accompany them to prenatal appointments or childbirth classes to alleviate their concerns.

Sleep Disturbances: Discomfort, frequent bathroom trips, and hormonal changes can disrupt sleep during pregnancy for partners as well. Help create a comfortable sleeping environment, offer massages or back rubs, and encourage relaxation techniques like deep breathing or meditation before bedtime.

Physical Discomforts: Partners may also experience physical discomforts such as back pain, headaches, and constipation. Offer assistance with household chores, encourage gentle exercises or stretches, and suggest alternative remedies like warm baths or prenatal massages.

Bonding with the Baby: Encourage partners to participate in activities that promote bonding with the baby, such as talking or singing to the bump, feeling for fetal movements, and attending prenatal classes together. Involve them in decision-making processes regarding the baby's nursery, clothing, and parenting philosophies.

Seeking Support: Remind partners that it's okay to seek support from friends, family members, or support groups if they're feeling overwhelmed or anxious about the pregnancy. Encourage open communication and assure them that their feelings are valid and normal.

By understanding and addressing the symptoms and challenges that partners may experience during pregnancy, you can provide invaluable support and strengthen your relationship as you navigate this transformative journey together.

Lifestyle changes: how to prepare for a healthy pregnancy

Preparing for a healthy pregnancy involves making lifestyle changes that support both the mother's well-being and the development of a healthy baby. Here's a comprehensive guide to help you prepare for a healthy pregnancy:

Preconception Health Check: Before conception, it's essential for both partners to undergo a preconception health check-up. This includes discussions with healthcare providers about medical history, current medications, vaccinations, and any pre-existing conditions that may impact pregnancy.

Nutrition: A balanced diet rich in fruits, vegetables, whole grains, lean proteins, and healthy fats is crucial for both partners. Prioritize foods high in folate, iron, calcium, and other essential nutrients. Consider taking prenatal vitamins containing folic acid before conception and throughout pregnancy to reduce the risk of neural tube defects.

Maintain a Healthy Weight: Aim for a healthy weight before conceiving, as being underweight or overweight can increase the risk of pregnancy complications. Incorporate regular exercise into your routine, such as walking, swimming, or prenatal yoga, to support overall health and well-being.

Avoid Harmful Substances: Eliminate or reduce exposure to harmful substances such as alcohol, tobacco, and recreational drugs, as they can negatively impact fertility and increase the risk of birth defects and pregnancy complications.

Manage Stress: Practice stress-reducing techniques such as mindfulness, meditation, deep breathing exercises, or yoga to promote emotional well-being and reduce the negative effects of stress on fertility and pregnancy.

Limit Caffeine Intake: Moderate caffeine consumption is generally considered safe during pregnancy, but excessive intake should be avoided. Limit caffeine intake to 200-300 milligrams per day, equivalent to about one 12-ounce cup of coffee.

Get Adequate Sleep: Prioritize getting enough sleep each night, aiming for 7-9 hours of quality rest. Create a comfortable sleep environment, establish a relaxing bedtime routine, and address any sleep disturbances or discomforts that may arise during pregnancy.

Stay Hydrated: To support optimal bodily functions, drink plenty of water throughout the day. Avoid sugary beverages and excessive caffeine intake, opting for water, herbal teas, and fresh fruit juices instead.

Practice Safe Sex: If you're trying to conceive, maintain a healthy sexual relationship with your partner and practice safe sex to prevent sexually transmitted infections (STIs) that can affect fertility and pregnancy outcomes.

Seek Prenatal Care: Schedule a preconception visit with a healthcare provider to discuss your plans for pregnancy and receive personalized guidance on optimizing your health and fertility. Once pregnant, attend regular prenatal appointments to monitor the progress of your pregnancy and address any concerns or complications that may arise.

By adopting these lifestyle changes and prioritizing
your health and well-being before and during
pregnancy, you can increase the likelihood of a
healthy conception, pregnancy, and delivery,
ultimately setting the stage for the well-being of
both you and your baby.

First time dads: tips and tricks[2]

For first-time dads, the journey into fatherhood can
be both exhilarating and daunting. Here are some
comprehensive tips and tricks to help navigate this
new role with confidence and support:

Educate Yourself: Learn about pregnancy,
childbirth, and newborn care. Attend prenatal
classes with your partner, read books, and seek
advice from experienced fathers or healthcare
professionals to better understand what to expect
during each stage of pregnancy and beyond.

Be Supportive: Pregnancy can be physically and
emotionally challenging for your partner. Be
supportive and attentive to her needs, offering help
with household chores, accompanying her to
appointments, and providing emotional
reassurance during times of stress or uncertainty.

Communicate Openly: Open and honest communication is key to building a strong foundation for your relationship as parents. Discuss your expectations, fears, and hopes for parenthood, and be willing to compromise and problem-solve together as a team.

Take Care of Yourself: Prioritize your own physical and mental well-being to be the best support system for your partner and baby. Make time for self-care activities such as exercise, hobbies, and socializing with friends to recharge and maintain a healthy balance in your life.

Bond with Your Baby: Start bonding with your baby even before birth by talking, singing, and reading to the bump. Attend prenatal appointments, feel for fetal movements, and participate in activities such as assembling the baby's nursery or choosing baby names to deepen your connection.

Prepare for Labor and Delivery: Familiarize yourself with the labor and delivery process, including different birthing techniques, pain management options, and your role as a birth partner. Be prepared to advocate for your partner's wishes and provide emotional support during labor and delivery.

Learn Newborn Care Skills: Take the time to learn practical newborn care skills such as diapering, bathing, feeding, and soothing techniques. Practice

hands-on caregiving tasks with a doll or by
assisting friends or family members with newborns
to build confidence and competence.

Be Flexible and Patient: Parenthood comes with its
fair share of surprises and challenges. Be flexible
and patient as you adjust to the demands of caring
for a newborn, and remember that it's okay to ask
for help or seek advice when needed.

Create a Support Network: Build a support network
of friends, family members, and fellow dads who
can offer guidance, encouragement, and practical
assistance along the way. Joining parenting groups
or online forums can also provide valuable
resources and camaraderie.

Celebrate Milestones: Cherish and celebrate each
milestone in your baby's development, from the first
smile to the first steps. Take plenty of photos and
create lasting memories as you embark on this
incredible journey of fatherhood.

By embracing these tips and tricks, first-time dads
can navigate the challenges and joys of parenthood
with confidence, love, and support for their partner
and new bundle of joy.

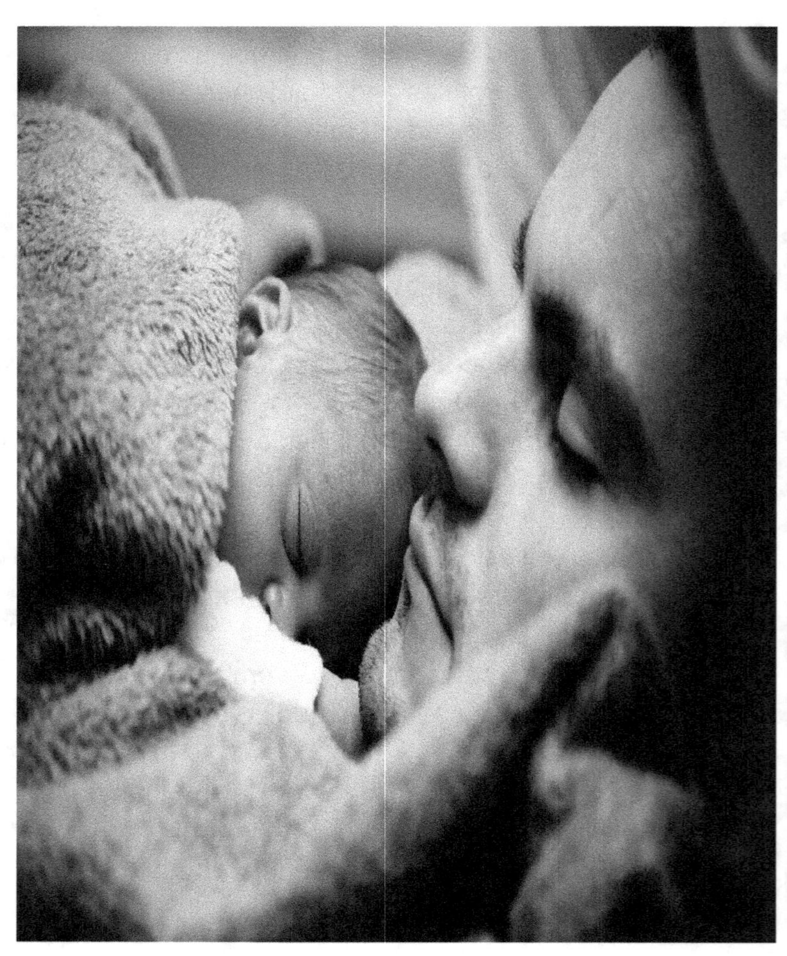

The Second Trimester

Baby development: what's happening during the second trimester

During the second trimester of pregnancy, which spans from weeks 13 to 27, significant developments occur in both the mother's body and the growing fetus. Here's a comprehensive overview:

1. Fetal Growth:

By the end of the first trimester, the fetus is approximately the size of a lime. By the end of the second trimester, it grows to around the size of a large banana.
Organs and body systems continue to develop and mature during this time. By the end of the second trimester, most of the baby's organs are formed and starting to function.

2. Facial Features:

The fetus's facial features become more defined. Eyebrows, eyelashes, and fingernails develop. The eyes, which initially formed at the end of the first trimester, can now blink.

3. Movements:

During the second trimester, the mother starts to feel fetal movements, commonly referred to as "quickening." These movements become more pronounced as the fetus grows and becomes stronger.

4. Vernix and Lanugo:

The fetus develops a protective coating called vernix caseosa, which covers its skin. This waxy substance helps protect the delicate skin from the amniotic fluid.
Fine hair called lanugo covers the fetus's body. This hair helps regulate the fetus's body temperature and usually sheds before birth.

5. Gender Identification:

In most cases, the sex of the baby can be determined during the second trimester through ultrasound imaging.

6. Maternal Changes:

The mother's abdomen starts to noticeably expand as the uterus grows to accommodate the growing fetus.

Many women experience relief from early pregnancy symptoms like nausea and fatigue during the second trimester, often referred to as the "honeymoon phase" of pregnancy.
Other symptoms may arise, such as backaches, constipation, and nasal congestion, as the body adjusts to the increasing size of the uterus and hormonal changes.
The mother may also experience emotional changes as the pregnancy progresses, ranging from excitement and anticipation to anxiety and mood swings.

7. Fetal Viability:

Towards the end of the second trimester, around week 24, the fetus reaches a stage of development where it may have a chance of survival outside the womb with medical intervention. This is known as fetal viability.

8. Diagnostic Tests:

During the second trimester, various diagnostic tests may be offered to monitor the health and development of the fetus, including ultrasound scans, amniocentesis, and maternal serum screening.

9. Bonding:

Many parents begin to feel a stronger emotional bond with their baby during the second trimester, as the pregnancy becomes more tangible with the mother's growing belly and the baby's movements being felt.
Overall, the second trimester is a period of significant growth and development for both the mother and the fetus, marked by noticeable physical changes and exciting milestones in the pregnancy journey.

Pregnancy symptoms: what your partner may experience and how to help

During pregnancy, partners may experience a range of symptoms and emotions as they navigate the journey alongside the pregnant person. Here's a comprehensive overview of common symptoms partners may experience and how to offer support:

1. Emotional Changes:

Partners may experience a rollercoaster of emotions, including excitement, anxiety, and mood swings. This is entirely normal and can be attributed to the significant life changes ahead.

How to help: Be patient, empathetic, and understanding. Listen actively to your partner's concerns and offer reassurance and support.

2. Physical Symptoms:

Some partners may experience physical symptoms similar to those of the pregnant person, albeit to a lesser extent. These symptoms can include fatigue, nausea, food cravings, and increased urination.
How to help: Offer practical support, such as taking on more household chores or preparing meals. Encourage your partner to rest when needed and accommodate any dietary preferences or aversions.

3. Weight Gain and Body Changes:

Partners may notice weight gain or changes in body shape, especially if they're actively involved in supporting their pregnant partner's dietary and lifestyle changes.
How to help: Offer positive reinforcement and avoid making comments about your partner's body unless they express a desire to discuss it. Encourage healthy habits, such as regular exercise and nutritious eating, for both of you.

4. Sleep Disturbances:

Sleep disruptions are common during pregnancy, and partners may also experience difficulty sleeping due to anxiety or discomfort.
How to help: Create a relaxing bedtime routine, minimize screen time before bed, and ensure the sleeping environment is comfortable. Consider using supportive pillows for better sleep quality.

5. Increased Stress and Responsibility:

Partners may feel added stress and responsibility as they anticipate the arrival of a new family member. This can manifest as worries about finances, parenting abilities, and relationship dynamics.
How to help: Communicate openly with your partner about your concerns and share the responsibilities of preparing for the baby's arrival. Attend prenatal appointments together and actively participate in decision-making processes.

6. Support During Labor and Delivery:

Partners may feel nervous or uncertain about their role during labor and delivery. They may worry about providing adequate support and being present for their partner during this intense experience.
How to help: Educate yourself about the labor and delivery process, attend childbirth classes together, and discuss your preferences and expectations

with your partner. Be a calming presence and offer physical and emotional support during labor.

7. Postpartum Adjustment:

The transition to parenthood can be challenging for both partners, and it's common to experience feelings of exhaustion, overwhelm, and uncertainty. How to help: Be proactive in supporting your partner's physical and emotional recovery after childbirth. Offer practical assistance with baby care tasks, encourage self-care, and seek support from family, friends, or a healthcare professional if needed.
Overall, supporting a pregnant partner involves being attentive, empathetic, and actively involved in their pregnancy journey. By offering practical assistance, emotional support, and open communication, partners can help alleviate some of the challenges and uncertainties associated with pregnancy and parenthood.

Gender reveal: how to find out and celebrate your baby's sex

Gender reveals have become popular ways for expectant parents to share the excitement of their baby's sex with family and friends. Here's a comprehensive guide on how to find out and celebrate your baby's sex:

1. Prenatal Screening:

The most common way to determine the sex of the baby is through prenatal screening, typically done through ultrasound imaging or non-invasive prenatal testing (NIPT).
Ultrasound scans are usually performed around 18-20 weeks gestation and can provide a clear view of the baby's anatomy, including their genitalia.
NIPT involves a blood test that analyzes fetal DNA in the mother's bloodstream to determine the baby's sex with a high level of accuracy. This test can be done as early as 10 weeks gestation.

2. Gender Reveal Parties:

Once the baby's sex has been determined, many parents choose to plan a gender reveal party to share the news with loved ones in a fun and creative way.
Popular gender reveal ideas include cutting into a cake filled with blue or pink frosting, releasing balloons or confetti in the corresponding color, or popping a balloon filled with colored powder.

3. Creative Gender Reveal Ideas:

Get creative with your gender reveal by incorporating themes or activities that reflect your interests and personalities as parents.

Some unique ideas include a sports-themed reveal with baseballs filled with colored powder, a "Waddle It Be?" rubber ducks floating in a pool of pink or blue water for a duck-themed reveal, or a "What's the Scoop? ice cream-themed reveal with blue or pink ice cream cones.

4. Social Media Announcements:

For those who prefer a more low-key approach, sharing the gender reveal on social media platforms like Instagram or Facebook can be a fun way to involve friends and family from afar. Consider posting a creative photo or video capturing the moment of the reveal, accompanied by a heartfelt caption expressing your excitement for your baby's arrival.

5. Inclusive Celebrations:

Keep in mind that gender reveals are optional, and not all expectant parents choose to participate. Some may prefer to wait until birth to find out the baby's sex or may opt for a more gender-neutral approach to parenting.
Regardless of how you choose to celebrate, focus on the joy and excitement of welcoming a new addition to your family, regardless of their gender.

6. Remember the Purpose:

While gender reveals can be a fun way to celebrate your baby's sex, it's essential to remember that gender is not synonymous with biological sex and may not fully encompass your child's identity.
As your child grows, they may express their gender in ways that challenge traditional norms, and it's essential to support and affirm their identity with love and acceptance.
Overall, gender reveals are a personal choice for expectant parents and can be a joyful way to celebrate the anticipation of welcoming a new baby into the world. Whether you choose a simple announcement or an elaborate party, the most important thing is to cherish the excitement and bond with loved ones as you prepare for this new chapter in your lives.

Baby shopping: what to buy and what to avoid

When it comes to baby shopping, it's easy to feel overwhelmed by the vast array of products available on the market. Here's a comprehensive guide on what to buy and what to avoid to help you navigate the process:

What to Buy:

Essential Clothing:

Invest in a variety of baby clothes, including onesies, sleepers, socks, hats, and mittens. Choose breathable, soft materials, like cotton, that are kind to your baby's sensitive skin.

Diapers and Wipes:

Stock up on diapers in various sizes, as well as baby wipes for diaper changes. Consider whether you prefer disposable or cloth diapers and choose accordingly.

Feeding Supplies:

If you're breastfeeding, consider purchasing a breast pump, nursing bras, nursing pads, and nipple cream. Bottles, nipples, formula (if not breastfeeding), and a bottle sterilizer are required for bottle-feeding.

Baby Gear:

Invest in essential baby gear such as a crib or bassinet, stroller, car seat, baby carrier or sling, and a diaper bag. Make sure these items meet safety standards and are appropriate for your lifestyle and budget.

Health and Safety Products:

Purchase a digital thermometer, infant nail clippers, baby grooming kit, baby monitor, and outlet covers to ensure your baby's health and safety.

Baby Bedding:

Buy fitted crib sheets, waterproof mattress covers, and lightweight blankets or sleep sacks to keep your baby comfortable and safe during sleep.

Baby Bathing Supplies:

Gather baby-friendly soap, shampoo, towels, washcloths, a bathtub or bathing seat, and a gentle baby brush for bath time.

Diapering Essentials:

Stock up on diaper rash cream, diaper pail liners, and a changing pad or table for convenient diaper changes.

Baby Toys and Entertainment:

Choose age-appropriate toys that stimulate your baby's senses and encourage development, such as rattles, soft plush toys, activity gyms, and board books.

What to Avoid:

Unnecessary Gadgets:

While there are many baby gadgets and devices on the market, not all of them are essential. Avoid purchasing unnecessary items that may clutter your home or drain your budget without providing significant benefits.

Unsafe Sleep Products:

Avoid purchasing crib bumpers, blankets, pillows, or stuffed animals for your baby's crib, as these items pose a suffocation hazard. Adhere to safe sleeping practices in order to lower the chance of SIDS.

Overstocking:

While it's tempting to buy everything you think you might need for your baby, try to avoid overstocking on items that may go unused. Babies grow quickly, and their needs may change over time, so it's okay to start with the essentials and add items as needed.

Single-Use Items:

Consider the longevity and versatility of items before purchasing. Single-use or short-lived products may not provide the best value for your money. Opt for multi-purpose items that can grow with your baby or serve multiple functions.
Non-Essential Baby Accessories:

While cute and trendy, some baby accessories like designer diaper bags or specialized baby clothing may not be worth the investment. Focus on practicality and functionality when choosing baby items.

Unsafe Products:

Avoid purchasing baby products that have been recalled or do not meet safety standards. Always research products thoroughly and read reviews before making a purchase to ensure they are safe and reliable for your baby.
By focusing on essential items that prioritize safety, comfort, and functionality, you can ensure a smooth and stress-free shopping experience as you prepare for the arrival of your little one. Remember to consider your budget, lifestyle, and personal preferences when making purchasing decisions, and don't hesitate to seek advice from experienced parents or healthcare professionals if you have any questions or concerns.

The Third Trimester

Baby development: what's happening during the third trimester

During the third trimester of pregnancy, which spans from week 28 until birth, remarkable developments occur in the baby's growth and organ maturation. Here's a comprehensive overview:

Size and Weight: The baby experiences a significant growth spurt, nearly doubling in weight from about 2.2 pounds (1 kg) at the beginning of the trimester to around 6.6 to 8.8 pounds (3 to 4 kg) at full term. The length also increases, with the average baby measuring around 19 to 22 inches (48 to 56 cm) by the end of the trimester.

Organ Development:

Brain: The brain continues to develop rapidly, with the cerebral cortex expanding and the brain structures becoming more complex.
Lungs: The lungs mature further, producing surfactant, a substance that helps the air sacs inflate and prevents them from collapsing after birth.

Liver and Kidneys: These organs become fully functional, aiding in metabolism and waste removal.
Digestive System: The digestive system is almost fully developed, with the intestines preparing to process breast milk or formula after birth.
Immune System: The immune system undergoes further development, acquiring antibodies from the mother to provide some immunity at birth.

Physical Features:

Hair and Nails: The baby's hair continues to grow, and the nails have usually reached the tips of the fingers.
Skin: The skin becomes less wrinkled as more fat accumulates beneath it, giving the baby a plumper appearance.
Skeletal System: Bones continue to harden, although the skull remains soft and flexible to facilitate passage through the birth canal.

Movement and Activity:

As space in the uterus becomes more limited, the baby's movements may feel different, with more rolling and stretching than kicking. However, the frequency of movements should remain consistent, indicating the baby's well-being.

Sensory Development:

The baby's senses, such as hearing and sight,
continue to develop. The baby can recognize
voices, sounds, and even some tastes from the
amniotic fluid.
Eyesight improves, although it remains blurry due
to the lack of light stimulation in the womb.

Positioning:

Towards the end of the trimester, most babies settle
into a head-down position in preparation for birth.
However, some babies may remain in a breech
(feet or buttocks first) or transverse (sideways)
position, requiring intervention or a cesarean
delivery.

Maturation of Body Systems:

The cardiovascular system continues to strengthen,
pumping more blood to support the growing body.
The endocrine system matures further, regulating
hormone production to maintain the pregnancy and
prepare for birth.

Fetal Development Monitoring:

Routine prenatal check-ups and ultrasound scans
are crucial during the third trimester to monitor the
baby's growth, position, and overall well-being.
These appointments also assess the mother's
health and readiness for childbirth.

Overall, the third trimester marks a period of rapid growth and development for the baby, preparing them for the transition to life outside the womb. It's a crucial time for both the baby and the mother as they anticipate the arrival of a new family member.

Pregnancy symptoms: what your partner may experience and how to help

During the third trimester of pregnancy, your partner may experience a range of physical and emotional symptoms as their body continues to adapt to the growing baby. Here's a comprehensive overview of common pregnancy symptoms and how you can help:

Physical Symptoms:

Fatigue: Your partner may feel more tired than usual, especially as the baby grows larger and puts more strain on their body. Encourage them to rest as needed and help out with household chores or errands to reduce their workload.
Backaches and Joint Pain: As the baby grows, the extra weight can strain your partner's back and joints. Offer massages or suggest prenatal yoga or gentle stretching exercises to alleviate discomfort.

Heartburn and Indigestion: Hormonal changes and the growing uterus can cause acid reflux and digestive issues. Encourage your partner to eat smaller, more frequent meals and avoid spicy or greasy foods.
Frequent Urination: Pressure on the bladder from the expanding uterus may lead to more frequent trips to the bathroom. Be patient and understanding if your partner needs to pause activities for bathroom breaks.
Swelling: Swelling in the feet, ankles, and hands, known as edema, is common in late pregnancy. Encourage your partner to elevate their feet when possible and avoid standing or sitting for long periods.
Shortness of Breath: As the uterus expands, it can push against the diaphragm and make breathing more difficult. Help your partner find comfortable positions for sleeping and relaxation, such as propping up pillows to elevate the upper body.
Braxton Hicks Contractions: These practice contractions may become more frequent and intense in the third trimester. Help your partner stay hydrated and encourage relaxation techniques to ease discomfort.

Emotional Symptoms:

Mood Swings: Hormonal changes, combined with the physical challenges of late pregnancy, can lead to mood swings and increased emotional sensitivity. Be patient and supportive, and listen to your partner's concerns without judgment.

Anxiety and Nervousness: As the due date approaches, your partner may feel anxious about labor, childbirth, and becoming a parent. Offer reassurance, attend prenatal classes together, and discuss any fears or concerns openly.

Nesting Instinct: Many expectant mothers experience a strong urge to prepare their home for the baby's arrival, known as the nesting instinct. Support your partner's nesting efforts by helping with tasks such as setting up the nursery or assembling baby furniture.

How to Help:

Provide Emotional Support: Be present, attentive, and empathetic to your partner's needs. Offer words of encouragement and reassurance, and actively listen to their thoughts and feelings.

Assist with Daily Tasks: Help with household chores, cooking, and running errands to alleviate your partner's physical burden and allow them more time to rest and relax.

Attend Prenatal Appointments: Accompany your partner to prenatal check-ups and ultrasounds to show your support and involvement in the pregnancy.

Educate Yourself: Take the time to learn about pregnancy, childbirth, and newborn care so you can better understand what your partner is experiencing and provide informed support.

Be Flexible and Understanding: Understand that your partner may have good days and bad days and be flexible with plans and expectations. Show understanding and patience during challenging moments.

By being attentive, supportive, and proactive, you can help ease your partner's discomfort and anxiety during the third trimester of pregnancy, strengthening your bond as you prepare for the arrival of your new family member.

Birth plan: how to prepare for labor and delivery

Preparing for labor and delivery involves creating a birth plan, gathering essential items, educating yourself about the process, and ensuring both physical and emotional readiness. Here's a comprehensive guide:

Create a Birth Plan:

Discuss your preferences with your partner, healthcare provider, and birth support team. Consider factors such as pain management options, delivery position preferences, and any special requests for the labor and delivery process.

Include contingency plans for unexpected situations, such as cesarean delivery or complications during labor.
Be flexible and open-minded, understanding that labor and delivery can be unpredictable.

Attend Prenatal Classes:

Enroll in prenatal classes to learn about childbirth, pain management techniques, breastfeeding, and newborn care.
Attend birthing classes together with your partner to understand each other's roles and responsibilities during labor and delivery.

Pack a Hospital Bag:

Pack essentials for labor, delivery, and postpartum recovery, including comfortable clothing, toiletries, snacks, a birth ball, massage tools, and items for relaxation.
Don't forget to include items for the baby, such as clothing, diapers, and blankets.

Stay Active and Healthy:

Engage in regular exercise and maintain a healthy diet to prepare your body for labor and recovery.
Practice relaxation techniques such as deep breathing, meditation, or prenatal yoga to manage stress and anxiety.

Communicate with Your Healthcare
Provider:

Discuss your birth plan with your healthcare
provider and address any concerns or questions
you may have.
Stay informed about the signs of labor and when to
contact your healthcare provider or go to the
hospital.

Prepare Your Support Team:

Communicate your birth plan and preferences with
your birth support team, including your partner,
doula, or other family members.
Discuss each person's role during labor and
delivery and ensure everyone is on the same page.

Create a Comfortable Environment:

Prepare your birthing environment by setting up a
calm and comfortable space at home or in the
hospital room.
Bring items that bring you comfort, such as music,
essential oils, or photos.

Stay Informed About Pain Management Options:

Explore different pain management techniques,
including medication, natural methods, and
relaxation techniques.

Discuss your preferences with your healthcare provider and keep an open mind about your options.

Know Your Rights and Advocacy:

Familiarize yourself with your rights as a patient and advocate for yourself during labor and delivery. Communicate your preferences and concerns with your healthcare team and ask questions if something is unclear or doesn't align with your wishes.

Emotional Preparation:

Prepare mentally and emotionally for labor and delivery by visualizing a positive birth experience and focusing on the end goal of meeting your baby. Seek support from your partner, friends, or a therapist if you're feeling anxious or overwhelmed about childbirth.
By taking proactive steps to prepare for labor and delivery, you can feel more confident and empowered as you approach the birth of your baby. Remember to stay flexible and open-minded, and trust in your body's ability to bring your baby into the world.

Hospital bag: what to pack and what to leave behind

When packing your hospital bag for labor and delivery, it's essential to include items that will keep you comfortable, prepared, and supported during this significant event. Here's a comprehensive list of what to pack and what you can leave behind:

Essentials for Labor and Delivery:

Medical Documents: Bring your ID, insurance information, and any necessary medical documents or birth plan.
Comfortable Clothing: Pack loose, comfortable clothing for labor, such as a nightgown, robe, or oversized T-shirt. Consider bringing clothes that are easy to move in and can accommodate monitoring devices.
Comfortable Shoes: Slip-on shoes or slippers that are easy to take on and off.
Toiletries: Include toiletries such as a toothbrush, toothpaste, shampoo, conditioner, body wash, and moisturizer. Don't forget hair ties or headbands.
Nursing Bra and Breast Pads: If you plan to breastfeed, pack a nursing bra and breast pads for comfort and leakage protection.
Maternity Pads: Bring maternity pads or adult diapers for postpartum bleeding.

Comfort Items: Bring items that provide comfort and relaxation, such as a pillow, blanket, massage tools, or essential oils.
Snacks: Pack snacks to keep your energy up during labor, such as granola bars, nuts, crackers, or fruit.
Hydration: Bring a water bottle or sports drink to stay hydrated during labor.
Entertainment: Consider bringing books, magazines, music, or a tablet with movies or TV shows to help pass the time during early labor.
Birth Ball: If you plan to use a birth ball for labor, consider bringing your own or checking if the hospital provides one.
Camera or Phone: Don't forget to bring a camera or smartphone to capture photos and videos of your baby's arrival.
Chargers: Bring chargers for your phone, camera, or any other electronic devices.
For Postpartum Recovery:

Comfortable Clothing: Pack comfortable, loose-fitting clothing for postpartum recovery, such as nursing-friendly tops, pajamas, and maternity leggings or sweatpants.
Toiletries: Continue to use your toiletries for postpartum hygiene, including items for showering and personal care.
Nursing Supplies: Bring nipple cream, nursing pads, and a breastfeeding pillow if you plan to breastfeed.

Postpartum Care Items: Pack items such as witch hazel pads, perineal spray, or a peri bottle for postpartum comfort.
Baby Clothes: Pack a few outfits for your baby, including onesies, sleepers, socks, and hats.
Car Seat: Make sure to install your baby's car seat correctly in your vehicle for the trip home.

What to Leave Behind:

Valuables: Leave valuables such as jewelry, expensive electronics, or large amounts of cash at home.
Unnecessary Items: Avoid bringing unnecessary items that will clutter your hospital room and be difficult to manage during labor and recovery.
Heavy Luggage: Keep your hospital bag lightweight and easy to carry, as you may need to move it around during labor and transport it to different areas of the hospital.
By packing thoughtfully and focusing on essentials, you can ensure that your hospital bag is well-prepared for labor, delivery, and postpartum recovery, while minimizing stress and unnecessary items.

The Birth

Labor signs: how to recognize and time contractions

Recognizing and timing contractions is crucial during labor to gauge the progression of childbirth and determine when to head to the hospital or birthing center. Here's a comprehensive guide:

Recognizing Labor Signs:
Contractions: These are the most common sign of labor. Contractions feel like intense menstrual cramps or tightening sensations in the lower abdomen or back.
Water Breaking: This can be a sudden gush or a slow trickle of amniotic fluid from the vagina. It may or may not be accompanied by contractions.
Bloody Show: This is when the mucus plug that sealed the cervix during pregnancy is expelled. It may be tinged with blood.
Cervical Changes: Your cervix may start to dilate (open) and efface (thin out). Your healthcare provider can check this during prenatal visits or during labor.
Timing Contractions:
Frequency: Contractions become regular and increasingly frequent as labor progresses. Initially, they may be irregular and spaced further apart.

Duration: Contractions typically last around 30 to 70 seconds in the early stages of labor but may lengthen as labor progresses.

Intensity: Contractions may start off mild and become stronger and more intense over time.

Location: Contractions often start in the lower back and move to the front of the abdomen as labor progresses.

How to Time Contractions:

Use a Timer: You can use a stopwatch, smartphone app, or contraction timing tool to track the duration and frequency of contractions.

Start Timing: Begin timing from the start of one contraction to the start of the next. Note the duration of each contraction and the time between them.

Keep Track: Record the duration and frequency of contractions on paper or digitally. This helps you and your healthcare provider monitor the progression of labor.

Stay Relaxed: Try to relax between contractions. Use deep breathing techniques or relaxation exercises to manage discomfort.

When to Call Your Healthcare Provider:

Regular Contractions: If contractions are consistently strong, last around 60 seconds or more, and occur every 5 minutes for at least an hour, contact your healthcare provider.

Water Breaking: Inform your healthcare provider if your water breaks, even if you're not experiencing contractions.

Decreased Fetal Movement: If you notice a significant decrease in fetal movement, contact your healthcare provider immediately.
Concerns or Questions: Don't hesitate to call your healthcare provider if you have any concerns or questions about labor signs or contractions.
Final Notes:
Every woman's labor experience is unique, so trust your instincts and seek medical advice if you're unsure.
Consider attending childbirth classes before labor to learn more about recognizing labor signs and coping techniques.
Have a plan in place for transportation to the hospital or birthing center once labor begins.

Stages of labor: what to expect and how to cope

Labor typically occurs in three main stages: the early stage, active stage, and transition stage. Here's a comprehensive guide on what to expect and how to cope with each stage:

1. Early Stage of Labor:
Duration: This stage can last for several hours or even days for some women.
Contractions: Contractions are typically mild to moderate and may feel like menstrual cramps.

They may start irregularly and become more regular over time.
Cervical Changes: Your cervix begins to dilate and efface (thin out).
What to Expect: You may experience excitement or anxiety as labor begins. Early labor is a good time to rest, eat light snacks, hydrate, and engage in relaxation techniques.
Coping Strategies:
Breathing Techniques: Practice slow, deep breathing to help manage discomfort and stay relaxed.
Movement: Walking, swaying, rocking, or changing positions can help ease pain and encourage the progress of labor. Massage: Applying mild counterpressure or massage to the lower back or abdomen can help relieve pain.
Warm Bath or Shower: Immersing in warm water can help soothe muscles and alleviate discomfort.

2. Active Stage of Labor:
Duration: This stage typically lasts from several hours to a few centimeters before full dilation.

Contractions: Contractions intensify and become more frequent, lasting around 60 to 90 seconds with shorter intervals between them.
Cervical Changes: Your cervix continues to dilate, usually reaching around 6 to 8 centimeters.
What to Expect: As labor progresses, you may feel more focused and determined. The intensity of

contractions increases, requiring more coping strategies.

Coping Strategies:
Focused Breathing: Practice focused breathing techniques, such as patterned breathing or rhythmic breathing, to manage pain and stay calm.

Position Changes: Experiment with different positions, such as standing, kneeling, squatting, or using a birthing ball, to find what's most comfortable.

Supportive Environment: Surround yourself with supportive birthing partners, healthcare providers, or a doula who can provide encouragement and comfort.
Hydration and Nutrition: Continue to stay hydrated with water or electrolyte drinks and consume light snacks to maintain energy levels.

3. Transition Stage of Labor:
Duration: This stage is the shortest but most intense phase of labor, typically lasting from a few minutes to an hour.
Contractions: Contractions are extremely intense, lasting around 60 to 90 seconds with very short breaks between them.
Cervical Changes: Your cervix completes dilation, reaching 10 centimeters.

What to Expect: Transition is often accompanied by intense emotions, including exhaustion, fear, and a strong urge to push.

Coping Strategies:
Focus and Visualization: Use visualization techniques to focus on the progress of labor and envision the birth of your baby.
Verbal Affirmations: Repeat positive affirmations or mantras to maintain confidence and motivation.

Encouragement: Lean on your support team for encouragement and reassurance during this challenging stage.
Pain Management Options: If desired, discuss pain management options with your healthcare provider, such as epidurals or nitrous oxide.

Final Notes:
Remember that every woman's labor experience is unique, and it's essential to find coping strategies that work best for you.
Communicate openly with your healthcare provider about your preferences for pain management and any concerns you may have during labor.
Stay flexible and be prepared to adapt your birth plan as labor progresses. Trust in your body's ability to give birth and seek support when needed.

Delivery options: pros and cons of natural, epidural, and cesarean birth

Each delivery option—natural birth, epidural, and cesarean section—has its own set of pros and cons. Here's an overview of each:

Natural Birth:
Pros:
Avoidance of Medications: Natural birth allows women to experience childbirth without the use of medications, which some women prefer for various reasons.
Mobility: Women giving birth naturally have the freedom to move around, change positions, and use gravity to aid in the birthing process.
Faster Recovery: Recovery time after a natural birth is typically quicker compared to other delivery methods, as there are no medications or surgical procedures involved.

Cons:
Pain: Labor pains can be intense and challenging to manage without medication, leading some women to find natural birth more uncomfortable.
Unpredictability: Labor can be unpredictable, and there's no guarantee of a smooth or complication-free delivery.

Potential for Intervention: In some cases, complications may arise during natural birth, necessitating medical intervention or emergency cesarean section.

Epidural:

Pros:
Pain Relief: Epidurals provide effective pain relief during labor, allowing women to experience childbirth with reduced discomfort.
Controlled Delivery: Epidurals allow women to remain awake and alert during delivery while managing pain effectively.
Reduced Stress: By minimizing pain and discomfort, epidurals can help reduce stress and anxiety during labor and delivery.

Cons:
Side Effects: Epidurals can cause side effects such as a drop in blood pressure, headache, shivering, or temporary loss of sensation in the lower body.
Restricted Mobility: Epidurals may limit mobility and the ability to change positions during labor, potentially prolonging the duration of labor.
Potential for Complications: While rare, epidurals can lead to complications such as nerve damage, infection, or allergic reactions.

Cesarean Birth:
Pros:

Controlled Environment: Cesarean births are planned surgical procedures, allowing for a controlled environment and predictable delivery.
Reduced Pain: Since cesarean births involve anesthesia, women typically experience less pain during the delivery process.
Prevention of Complications: In some cases, cesarean birth may be necessary to prevent complications for the mother or baby, such as fetal distress or placenta previa.

Cons:
Recovery Time: Recovery after a cesarean birth typically takes longer compared to vaginal delivery, involving post-surgical care and restrictions on physical activity.
Risk of Complications: Cesarean births carry a higher risk of complications such as infection, blood loss, blood clots, and injury to organs.
Impact on Future Pregnancies: Multiple cesarean births may increase the risk of complications in future pregnancies, including placental abnormalities and uterine rupture.

Final Considerations:
The choice of delivery method depends on individual preferences, medical considerations, and the recommendations of healthcare providers.
It's essential for expectant mothers to discuss their birth preferences and concerns with their healthcare team to make informed decisions about

the best delivery option for their unique
circumstances.
Regardless of the chosen delivery method, the
primary goal is a safe and healthy outcome for both
mother and baby.

Birth partner role: how to support your partner and meet your baby

Support from a birth partner plays a crucial role in
the birthing process, providing emotional, physical,
and practical assistance to the laboring mother.
Here's a comprehensive guide on how to support
your partner and welcome your baby into the world:

Before Labor:
Attend Prenatal Classes: Accompany your partner
to prenatal classes to learn about the birthing
process, comfort measures, and techniques for
labor support.
Discuss Birth Preferences: Have open and honest
discussions with your partner about her birth
preferences, including pain management options,
birthing environment, and any concerns or fears
she may have.
Create a Birth Plan: Work together to create a birth
plan that outlines your preferences for labor and
delivery, including preferences for pain
management, interventions, and postpartum care.

Pack a Hospital Bag: Help your partner pack a hospital bag with essentials for labor and postpartum recovery, including comfortable clothing, toiletries, snacks, and entertainment.

During Labor:
Provide Emotional Support: Offer words of encouragement, reassurance, and love to your partner throughout labor. Remind her of her strength and the progress she's making.
Physical Comfort Measures: Use massage, counter-pressure, and relaxation techniques to help alleviate discomfort during contractions. Assist your partner in finding comfortable positions and provide physical support as needed.
Keep Her Hydrated and Nourished: Offer water, ice chips, and light snacks to keep your partner hydrated and maintain her energy levels during labor.

Advocate for Her Needs: Communicate with healthcare providers on behalf of your partner, ensuring that her wishes and preferences are respected and addressed during labor and delivery.
Maintain a Calm Environment: Create a calm and supportive environment in the birthing room, dimming lights, playing soothing music, and minimizing distractions to help your partner feel relaxed and focused.
Be Flexible: Be prepared to adapt to changes in the birth plan or unexpected circumstances during

labor, offering flexibility and support to your partner as needed.

Welcoming Your Baby:
Be Present and Engaged: Stay by your partner's side during the birth of your baby, offering emotional support and encouragement as she pushes.
Prepare for Skin-to-Skin Contact: After birth, facilitate skin-to-skin contact between your partner and the baby to promote bonding and regulate the baby's temperature and breathing.

Assist with Breastfeeding: Help your partner with breastfeeding by offering support, positioning assistance, and encouragement. Attend breastfeeding classes together to learn about proper latch and breastfeeding techniques.
Share Responsibilities: Take an active role in caring for your newborn, including diaper changes, soothing, and bonding activities. Share responsibilities with your partner to ensure both of you have time to rest and recover.

Capture Memories: Take photos and videos to capture precious moments during the birth of your baby, creating lasting memories for your family.
After Labor:
Offer Postpartum Support: Be attentive to your partner's needs during the postpartum period, offering emotional support, practical assistance,

and encouragement as she recovers from childbirth.

Communicate Openly: Keep communication lines open with your partner, discussing any concerns, challenges, or adjustments you may be experiencing as new parents.

Seek Help if Needed: Encourage your partner to seek help from healthcare providers, lactation consultants, or support groups if she's experiencing postpartum mood disorders or breastfeeding difficulties.

Celebrate Your New Family: Take time to celebrate the arrival of your baby and the new chapter in your lives as a family. Cherish the moments together and express gratitude for the support and love you share.

By actively participating in the birthing process and providing unwavering support to your partner, you play an invaluable role in creating a positive and memorable birth experience for both your partner and your baby.

The Fourth Trimester

Baby care: how to feed, change, bathe, and soothe your newborn

The fourth trimester refers to the first three months after a baby is born, during which both the baby and the parents are adjusting to life outside the womb. During this period, newborns are adjusting to the world around them, and parents are learning how to care for their new addition. Here's a comprehensive guide on baby care during the fourth trimester:

Feeding:

Breastfeeding: A newborn's best source of nutrition is breast milk. It provides essential nutrients and antibodies that help protect the baby from infections. Newborns should breastfeed frequently, about every 2-3 hours, or whenever they show signs of hunger.
Formula feeding: If breastfeeding is not possible, formula feeding is a good alternative. Formula-fed babies typically eat every 3-4 hours, and parents should follow the instructions on the formula packaging for proper preparation.

Changing:

Diaper changing: Newborns typically need their diapers changed 8-12 times a day. To avoid diaper rash, it's critical to maintain a dry and clean diaper area. Use mild wipes or water and cotton balls for cleaning, and apply a diaper cream to protect the skin.

Umbilical cord care: Until the umbilical cord stump falls off (usually within 1-2 weeks), keep the area clean and dry. Fold diapers below the stump to avoid irritation, and avoid giving baths until the stump falls off.

Bathing:

Sponge baths: Until the umbilical cord stump falls off, give your newborn sponge baths using a soft washcloth and warm water. Gently wash the baby's face, body, and diaper area, being careful around the umbilical cord stump.

Tub baths: Once the umbilical cord stump falls off, you can start giving your baby tub baths. Use a baby bathtub or a sink filled with a few inches of warm water. Support the baby's head and neck, and never leave them unattended in the water.

Soothing:

Swaddling: Wrapping your baby snugly in a blanket can help them feel secure and calm. Make sure the swaddle is not too tight and that the baby's hips can move freely.

Sucking: Sucking is a natural reflex for babies and can help soothe them. Offer a pacifier or let them nurse for comfort.

Skin-to-skin contact: Holding your baby against your bare chest can help regulate their temperature, heart rate, and breathing, and promote bonding.

Rocking and motion: Gently rocking or swaying your baby in your arms or a rocking chair can help calm them down.

White noise: Soft, rhythmic sounds like a fan, white noise machine, or even a vacuum cleaner can help soothe a fussy baby by mimicking the sounds they heard in the womb.

Remember, every baby is unique, so it may take some trial and error to figure out what works best for soothing your newborn. Trust your instincts and don't hesitate to ask for help from healthcare professionals or experienced parents if you need it.

Postpartum recovery: what your partner may experience and how to help

Postpartum recovery is not only a physical process for the mother but also a significant transition period for the partner. Here's a comprehensive guide on what your partner may experience during postpartum recovery and how you can help:

Physical Changes:

Fatigue: Your partner may experience exhaustion due to disrupted sleep patterns, nighttime feedings, and the physical demands of caring for a newborn.
Hormonal Changes: Just like the mother, partners may experience hormonal shifts postpartum, which can lead to mood swings, irritability, or feelings of sadness.
Increased Responsibilities: Partners may take on additional household tasks, such as cooking, cleaning, and running errands, to support the mother during her recovery.

Emotional Changes:

Anxiety: Partners may feel anxious about their new role as a parent, concerns about the baby's well-being, or worries about providing for their growing family.
Bonding: While some partners may feel an instant bond with their newborn, others may take more time to develop a strong connection. This is normal and can be influenced by factors such as the birth experience, stress, and fatigue.
Supporting the Mother: Partners may feel pressure to be the primary source of support for the mother, which can be emotionally taxing, especially if they are also experiencing their own challenges.

How to Help:

Encourage Self-Care: Encourage your partner to prioritize self-care activities, such as taking breaks, getting enough rest, and engaging in activities they enjoy.

Share Responsibilities: Take an active role in caring for the baby and managing household tasks. Offer to change diapers, feed the baby, and take over nighttime duties to give your partner a chance to rest.

Listen and Validate: Be a supportive listener and offer validation for your partner's feelings and experiences. Tell them you are here to support them and that you understand that their feelings are legitimate.

Provide Affection: Offer physical affection and emotional support to reassure your partner of your love and appreciation. Simple gestures like hugs, kisses, and words of encouragement can make a big difference.

Seek Help if Needed: Encourage your partner to seek professional help if they are struggling with postpartum depression or anxiety. Offer to accompany them to therapy sessions or doctor's appointments for support.

Remember that postpartum recovery is a journey for both partners, and open communication, empathy, and mutual support are key to navigating this period together. By working as a team and prioritizing each other's well-being, you can strengthen your relationship and adapt to your new roles as parents.

Parenting challenges: how to deal with sleep deprivation, colic, and crying

Parenting challenges such as sleep deprivation, colic, and excessive crying can be overwhelming for new parents. Here's a comprehensive guide on how to deal with each of these challenges:

Sleep Deprivation:

Establish a Routine: Create a consistent bedtime routine for your baby, including activities like bathing, feeding, and bedtime stories. You can help your baby learn when it's time to go to sleep by being consistent.
Take Turns: Share nighttime responsibilities with your partner. Take turns soothing the baby, changing diapers, and feeding to ensure that both parents get adequate rest.
Maximize Daytime Sleep: Encourage naps during the day to help make up for lost sleep at night. Create a calm and quiet environment for daytime sleep, and consider babywearing or using a stroller for naps on the go.
Accept Help: Don't hesitate to accept help from family and friends. Allow loved ones to assist with household chores, meal preparation, or childcare so that you can prioritize rest.
Colic:

Comfort Measures: Try various comfort measures to soothe your baby during colicky episodes, such as gentle rocking, swaddling, or using a pacifier. Experiment with different holding positions to find what works best for your baby.

White Noise: Background noise, such as a fan, vacuum cleaner, or white noise machine, can help mask external stimuli and provide a calming effect for colicky babies.

Gas Relief: If gas is contributing to your baby's discomfort, try gentle tummy massage, bicycle leg movements, or using over-the-counter gas drops as directed by your pediatrician.

Seek Support: Join a support group for parents of colicky babies to connect with others who are going through similar experiences. Sharing tips and coping strategies with other parents can provide valuable support and reassurance.

Excessive Crying:

Check for Basic Needs: Ensure that your baby's basic needs, such as hunger, thirst, diaper change, and comfort, are met. Sometimes excessive crying can be a sign of discomfort or illness.

Comfort and Soothe: Use gentle rocking, swaying, or rhythmic movements to comfort your baby. Skin-to-skin contact, gentle massage, and soft singing or humming can also help soothe a crying baby.

Take Breaks: If you find yourself becoming overwhelmed by your baby's crying, it's okay to

take a short break. Place your baby in a safe
space, such as a crib or bassinet, and step away
for a few minutes to collect yourself.
Consult Your Pediatrician: If your baby's crying
persists or if you're concerned about their
well-being, don't hesitate to consult your
pediatrician. They can rule out any underlying
medical issues and provide guidance on managing
excessive crying.
Remember that parenting challenges are
temporary, and it's okay to ask for help when you
need it. Be patient with yourself and your baby, and
trust that you'll find effective strategies for
managing these challenges over time.

Relationship changes: how to keep the romance alive and communicate effectively

Maintaining a strong and romantic relationship after
having a baby can be challenging, but with effort
and communication, it's possible to keep the spark
alive. Here's a guide on how to keep the romance
alive and communicate effectively in your
relationship:

Keeping the Romance Alive:

Schedule Quality Time: Make time for each other by scheduling regular date nights or couple activities. Even if it's just a quiet evening at home after the baby is asleep, prioritize spending quality time together.

Express Appreciation: Show appreciation for your partner's efforts, whether it's helping with childcare, managing household tasks, or simply being supportive. Small gestures of gratitude can go a long way in strengthening your bond.

Physical Affection: Don't underestimate the power of physical touch. Hug, kiss, and cuddle with your partner regularly to maintain intimacy and connection.

Surprise Gestures: Surprise your partner with thoughtful gestures, such as love notes, small gifts, or acts of service. These unexpected acts of kindness can reignite the romance in your relationship.

Open Communication: Keep the lines of communication open and honest. Share your thoughts, feelings, and concerns with each other, and be receptive to your partner's perspective.

Spice Things Up: Explore new experiences together to keep things exciting. Try new hobbies, travel to new places, or experiment with different activities in the bedroom to keep the passion alive.

Communicating Effectively:

Active Listening: Show your partner that you are paying close attention to them when they are speaking. Ask clarifying questions to make sure you understand, and refrain from interrupting or making snap judgments.

Use "I" Statements: When expressing your thoughts or feelings, use "I" statements to avoid blaming or accusing your partner. For example, say "I feel..." instead of "You always..."

Validate Feelings: Validate your partner's feelings and experiences, even if you don't necessarily agree with them. Let them know that their emotions are valid and that you're there to support them.

Compromise: Be willing to compromise and find solutions that work for both of you. Focus on finding common ground rather than trying to "win" arguments.

Manage Conflict: Approach conflict with a calm and respectful attitude. Take breaks if emotions escalate, and come back to the discussion when you're both in a more rational state of mind.

Seek Professional Help: If communication issues persist or if you're struggling to resolve conflicts on your own, consider seeking couples therapy or counseling. A trained therapist can provide guidance and tools to improve communication and strengthen your relationship.

Recall that it requires work on the part of both partners to keep a relationship strong. By prioritizing communication, expressing love and appreciation, and making time for each other, you can keep the romance alive and build a strong foundation for your family.

CONCLUSION

In conclusion, navigating the journey of pregnancy as a first-time dad can be both exhilarating and challenging. By actively engaging in education, support, and communication with your partner, you can play an integral role in the pregnancy experience. Remember to prioritize empathy, patience, and flexibility as you embark on this transformative journey together. Ultimately, embracing the responsibilities and joys of impending fatherhood will not only strengthen your relationship but also lay the foundation for a fulfilling and supportive family dynamic for years to come.

The joys and struggles of parenthood

Parenthood is a rich tapestry woven with both joys and struggles. The joys are abundant and diverse, from the unparalleled love and bond shared with your child to the simple yet profound moments of laughter and discovery. Witnessing your child's first smile, hearing their infectious laughter, and celebrating their milestones fill your heart with an indescribable sense of fulfillment.

However, there are challenges associated with being a parent as well. The sleepless nights, the constant juggling of responsibilities, and the worry that accompanies every decision can be overwhelming at times. Balancing work, family, and personal needs requires patience, resilience, and adaptation.

Despite the challenges, parenthood offers invaluable lessons in patience, selflessness, and unconditional love. It teaches us to find joy in the little things, appreciate the beauty of imperfection, and cherish the fleeting moments that make up our children's childhood.

In the end, the joys of parenthood far outweigh the struggles. The profound connection forged with your child, the growth and development witnessed firsthand, and the profound sense of purpose that comes with nurturing another life make every sacrifice worthwhile. Parenthood is a journey filled with ups and downs, but it's a journey that transforms us in ways we never thought possible.

Resources and advice for new dads

For new dads embarking on the journey of fatherhood, there are numerous resources and advice available to help navigate this exciting and sometimes overwhelming transition. Here's a guide:

Books: There are many books tailored specifically for new dads. Some popular titles include "The Expectant Father" by Armin A. Brott and Jennifer Ash, "Dude, You're Gonna Be a Dad!" by John Pfeiffer, and "Fatherhood: The Ultimate Guide" by Armin A. Brott. These books cover everything from pregnancy and childbirth to newborn care and parenting tips.

Online Communities: Joining online forums and communities for dads can provide invaluable support and advice. Websites like Daddit (on Reddit), DadLabs, and The Dad Website offer forums, articles, and resources tailored for fathers.

Parenting Classes: Consider enrolling in parenting classes, either in person or online. Many hospitals and community centers offer classes specifically designed for expectant fathers, covering topics such as childbirth, newborn care, and parenting skills.

Support Groups: Seek out local support groups or meetups for new dads. Connecting with other fathers who are going through similar experiences can provide a sense of camaraderie and validation. These groups often offer opportunities to share tips, ask questions, and receive support.

Online Resources: Explore reputable websites and blogs dedicated to fatherhood and parenting. Websites like Fatherly, The Dad, and The Art of Manliness offer articles, videos, and resources on a wide range of parenting topics, from pregnancy and childbirth to father-child bonding and beyond.

Apps: There are several apps designed to support new dads throughout the parenting journey. Apps like DaddyUp, BabyCenter's My Baby Today, and Baby Tracker: Newborn Log offer tools for tracking diaper changes, feedings, sleep patterns, and developmental milestones, as well as providing helpful tips and advice.

Talk to Other Dads: Don't hesitate to reach out to other fathers in your life – whether it's your own father, friends who are dads, or colleagues. Their firsthand experiences and advice can be incredibly valuable as you navigate the ups and downs of fatherhood.

Self-Care: Remember to prioritize self-care as you adjust to your new role as a dad. Taking care of your physical and mental well-being is crucial for being the best parent you can be. Find time for hobbies, exercise, and relaxation, and don't be afraid to ask for help when you need it.

By utilizing these resources and seeking support from fellow dads, you can feel more confident and prepared as you embrace the joys and challenges of fatherhood. Remember, no one has all the answers, and it's okay to make mistakes – what matters most is your love, dedication, and commitment to being the best dad you can be.

Congratulations on becoming a dad!!

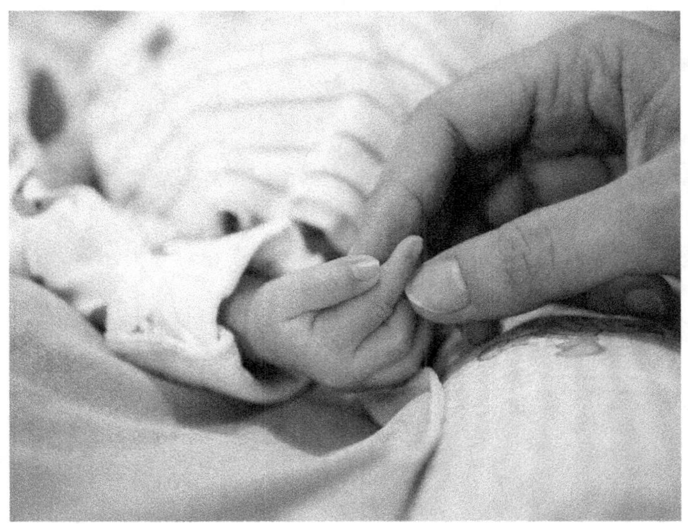